The Ultimate guide to longevity and good health

How to live a healthy longlife

Anthony J. Janes

Table of contents

Introduction

Welcome to "The Ultimate Guide to Longevity and Good Health" - a book that will take you on a journey to discover the secrets of living a long, healthy and fulfilling life. In today's fast-paced world, where stress, pollution, and unhealthy lifestyles have become the norm, it's more important than ever to take care of our health and wellbeing.

In this book, you will learn about the latest scientific research and time-tested practices that can help you improve your health and increase your lifespan. From nutrition and exercise to sleep and stress management, this guide covers all the essential aspects of living a healthy life.

But this is not just another health book. "The Ultimate Guide to Longevity and Good Health" is a comprehensive and practical guide that will help you make real, sustainable changes in your life. You will find easy-to-follow tips, practical advice, and much more that will motivate you to take charge of your health and live your best life.

Whether you are young or old, healthy or struggling with a health condition, this book is for you. So, get ready to embark on a journey to discover the secrets of longevity and good health - and start living your best life today!

Quotes on Health and longevity

"The first wealth is health." - Ralph Waldo Emerson

"A healthy outside starts from the inside." - Robert Urich

"Take care of your body, it's the only place you have to live." - Jim Rohn

"The greatest wealth is health." - Virgil

"Health is a state of complete harmony of the body, mind, and spirit." - B.K.S. Iyengar

"Investing in your health is the best investment you can make." - Bethenny Frankel

"To keep the body in good health is a duty... otherwise, we shall not be able to keep our mind strong and clear." - Buddha

"Longevity is a sign of a well-lived life." - Joseph B. Wirthlin

"Longevity is not just about living long, but about living well." - Dan Buettner

"The key to longevity is to learn every aspect of your being, and then take control of your health." - Deepak Chopra

"Longevity is not a matter of age; it is a matter of vitality." - Stephen Cherniske

"The secret to a long and healthy life is to be stress-free. Be grateful for everything you have, stay away from people who are negative, stay smiling and keep running." - Fauja Singh

Chapter One

Nutrition and Lifestyle habits.

The importance of a healthy and balanced diet to living a longlife cannot be overemphasized.

Maintaining a healthy and balanced diet is one of the most important factors for living a long and healthy life. Below are some reasons why we need a healthy and balanced diet for longevity.

- Reducing the risk of chronic diseases: A healthy diet can help reduce the risk of chronic diseases such as heart disease, diabetes, and certain types of cancer. Eating a variety of nutrient-rich foods such as fruits, vegetables, whole grains, lean proteins, and healthy fats can help provide the body with the necessary nutrients it needs to function properly and reduce the risk of these diseases.

- Maintaining a healthy weight: A healthy diet can help maintain a healthy weight, which is crucial for overall health and longevity. Eating a balanced diet that is low in processed and high-calorie foods can help prevent obesity and related health problems.

- Boosting the immune system: A healthy diet can help boost the immune system, which is essential for fighting off infections and diseases. Nutrient-rich foods such as fruits, vegetables, and whole grains contain vitamins and minerals that can help support the immune system.

- Improving mental health: A healthy diet can also have a positive impact on mental health. Eating a diet that is rich in whole foods and low in processed foods has been linked to a lower risk of depression and anxiety.

In summary, a healthy and balanced diet is crucial for living a long and healthy life. It can help reduce the risk of chronic diseases, maintain a healthy weight, boost the immune system, and improve mental health.

Another issue to critically consider when it comes to living long is the benefits of whole foods.

Whole foods can provide numerous benefits to living a long life, some of these benefits are explained below.

- Nutrient density: Whole foods are typically nutrient-dense, meaning they provide a high concentration of essential vitamins, minerals, and other nutrients that are necessary for overall health and longevity.

- Fiber: Whole foods are also high in fiber, which can promote digestive health and help regulate blood sugar levels, reducing the risk of chronic diseases such as diabetes, heart disease, and certain types of cancer.

- Antioxidants: Many whole foods are rich in antioxidants, which can help protect against cellular damage caused by free radicals, reducing the risk of chronic diseases associated with aging.

- Anti-inflammatory properties: Whole foods can also have anti-inflammatory properties, which can help reduce inflammation in the body, a key contributor to many chronic diseases.

- Low in additives and preservatives: Whole foods are typically minimally processed and do not contain added sugars, preservatives, or other artificial ingredients, which can have negative health effects over time.

- Support healthy weight: Eating whole foods can help maintain a healthy weight, reducing the risk of obesity-related diseases such as diabetes, heart disease, and certain cancers.

Without mincing words, incorporating whole foods into your diet can help promote optimal health and longevity.

However, what we should not ignore when dealing with health and long life is the dangers of processed foods and sugar.

Processed foods and sugar are commonly consumed in today's modern diet, but they pose significant dangers to good health and long life. Below are some notable reasons why they are not in alignment with good health and long life.

- Obesity: Processed foods and sugary drinks are high in calories and low in nutrients, leading to weight gain and obesity. Obesity is a major risk factor for numerous chronic diseases, including heart disease, diabetes, and certain types of cancer.

- Diabetes: A diet high in processed foods and sugar can increase the risk of developing type 2 diabetes. When you consume too much sugar, your body produces more insulin, which can eventually lead to insulin resistance, a key factor in the development of diabetes.

- Heart disease: Processed foods are often high in unhealthy fats, sodium, and added sugars, which can lead to high blood pressure, high cholesterol,

and other risk factors for heart
disease.

- Inflammation: Processed foods and
sugar can cause chronic inflammation
in the body, which is linked to a wide
range of health problems, including
autoimmune diseases, cancer, and
depression.

- Nutrient deficiencies: Processed foods
often lack essential nutrients, such as
fiber, vitamins, and minerals, that are
needed for good health. This can lead
to nutrient deficiencies and a higher
risk of chronic disease.

- Addiction: Processed foods and sugar
can be addictive, leading to cravings

and overconsumption. This can make it difficult to maintain a healthy diet and can lead to long-term health problems.

- Increased risk of cancer: A diet high in processed foods and sugar has been linked to an increased risk of certain types of cancer, including colon cancer, breast cancer, and pancreatic cancer.

In conclusion, consuming processed foods and sugar on a regular basis can have serious negative impacts on your health, increasing your risk of numerous chronic diseases and lowering your life expectancy. A diet rich in whole, unprocessed foods, and low in sugar is recommended for good health and a longer life.

Lifestyle habits

Your continual habits like smoking, excessive alcohol consumption, and drug use amongst others, could endanger your health and in the long run your lifespan.

Negative lifestyle habits such as smoking, excessive alcohol consumption, and drug use can have a significant impact on your health and well-being, both in the short term and the long run. These habits can lead to a range of health problems, including chronic diseases, mental health issues, and premature death. Below are some of the ways these habits can endanger your health and lifespan.

- Smoking: Smoking is one of the most dangerous and common negative lifestyle habits. It can lead to a range of health problems, including lung cancer, heart disease, stroke, and respiratory illnesses like chronic obstructive pulmonary disease (COPD). Smoking also damages the immune system, making you more susceptible to infections and diseases. According to the World Health Organization (WHO), tobacco use is responsible for approximately 8 million deaths each year worldwide, and this number is expected to increase in the future.

- Excessive alcohol consumption: Drinking too much alcohol can also lead to a range of health problems, including liver disease, high blood pressure, heart disease, and certain types of cancer. Excessive drinking can also lead to mental health issues such as depression and anxiety. According to the National Institute on Alcohol Abuse and Alcoholism, alcohol-related deaths in the United States alone reached nearly 95,000 in 2020.

- Drug use: The use of illegal drugs or even some prescription drugs can have significant negative effects on your health. Drug use can lead to addiction, overdose, and even death. Many drugs can damage your organs, including your liver, kidneys, and brain. Additionally, drug use can lead to mental health issues such as anxiety, depression, and psychosis.

In a nutshell, negative lifestyle habits such as smoking, excessive alcohol consumption, and drug use can have significant negative effects on your health and lifespan. These habits increase your risk of developing chronic diseases, mental health issues, and can lead to premature death. It is essential to take steps to reduce or eliminate these habits to improve your health and longevity.

Chapter Two

Exercise, Sleep and Stress management.

The benefits of regular physical activity to health and longlife cannot be overemphasized.

Regular physical activities has been shown to have numerous benefits for living a long and healthy life. Explained below are some of the key benefits.

- Reducing the risk of chronic diseases: Regular physical activity can help prevent or manage chronic diseases such as heart disease, stroke, type 2 diabetes, and certain types of cancer. This can significantly improve overall health and increase lifespan.

- Maintaining a healthy weight: Regular physical activity can help maintain a healthy weight, which in turn reduces the risk of chronic diseases.

- Strengthening bones and muscles: Regular physical activity helps to strengthen bones and muscles, reducing the risk of fractures and falls, especially in older adults.

- Improving mental health: Regular physical activity can help reduce stress, anxiety, and depression, and improve overall mood and well-being.

- Improving sleep: Regular physical activity can improve the quality of sleep, leading to increased energy levels and improved overall health.

- Improving cognitive function: Regular physical activity has been shown to improve cognitive function and reduce the risk of cognitive decline in older adults.

Conclusively, regular physical activity is a key component of a healthy lifestyle and can significantly improve quality of life and increase lifespan. It is recommended that adults engage in at least 150 minutes of moderate-intensity aerobic physical activity or 75 minutes of vigorous-intensity aerobic physical activity per week, as well as muscle-strengthening activities at least two days per week

Cardiovascular health: This is primarily concerned with the heart and the blood vessels. However, the concept of sleep, exercise and stress management can help to improve cardiovascular health.

Benefits of improved cardiovascular health to longlife.

Improved cardiovascular health can have a significant positive impact on long life. Below are some of the benefits of improved cardiovascular health to long life:

- Reduced risk of heart disease: Heart disease is the leading cause of death worldwide. Improving your cardiovascular health can significantly reduce your risk of developing heart disease, which can help you live a longer, healthier life.

- Lower blood pressure: High blood pressure is a major risk factor for heart disease and other health problems. Improving your cardiovascular health can help lower your blood pressure, reducing your risk of developing related health problems.

- Improved circulation: Good cardiovascular health promotes good circulation, which helps deliver oxygen and nutrients to your cells and tissues. This can help keep your body healthy and functioning properly.

- Reduced risk of stroke: Stroke is another leading cause of death worldwide. Improving your cardiovascular health can significantly reduce your risk of developing a stroke, which can help you live a longer, healthier life.

- Better overall health: Good cardiovascular health is closely linked to good overall health. Improving your cardiovascular health can help you feel better, have more energy, and reduce your risk of developing other health problems.

In the long run, improving your cardiovascular health can have a profound positive impact on your long life. By reducing your risk of heart disease, stroke, and other health problems, you can live a longer, healthier life with improved quality of life.

Weight control: This also enhances good health and life span. And it can be achieved via the process of exercise, sleep amongst others.

Maintaining a healthy weight can have numerous benefits for overall health and longevity. Here are a few ways weight control can enhance living long.

- Reduces the risk of chronic diseases: Being overweight or obese is linked to an increased risk of many chronic diseases, such as heart disease, diabetes, and certain cancers. By maintaining a healthy weight, you can lower your risk of developing these conditions and improve your chances of living a longer, healthier life.

- Improves cardiovascular health: Carrying excess weight puts extra strain on the heart and blood vessels, which can lead to high blood pressure, high cholesterol, and other cardiovascular problems. By maintaining a healthy weight, you can reduce your risk of developing these conditions and improve the health of your heart and blood vessels.

- Increases mobility and independence: Carrying excess weight can make it more difficult to move around and perform everyday tasks. By maintaining a healthy weight, you can improve your mobility and independence, which can enhance your quality of life as you age.

- Improves mental health: Being overweight or obese can also have a negative impact on mental health, leading to issues such as depression and anxiety. By maintaining a healthy weight, you can improve your self-esteem and overall sense of well-being.

Without mincing matters, weight control is an important factor in living a long and healthy life. By maintaining a healthy weight through a balanced diet and regular exercise, you can reduce your risk of chronic diseases, improve your cardiovascular health, increase your mobility and independence, and enhance your mental health.

Some golden facts about getting enough quality sleep.

- Getting enough quality sleep is essential for maintaining good health and longevity. During sleep, the body performs critical restorative and repair functions, including consolidating memories, repairing tissues, and regulating hormones.

- When you get enough high-quality sleep, you are more likely to have a better mood, increased productivity, and improved cognitive function. In contrast, lack of sleep or poor sleep quality can lead to a range of negative health outcomes, including increased risk of chronic conditions such as obesity, diabetes, and heart disease.

- Research has shown that sleep plays a crucial role in the immune system, and getting enough quality sleep helps to support the body's ability to fight off infection and disease. Furthermore, a good night's sleep is associated with better emotional regulation, stress management, and overall mental health.

In conclusion, getting enough quality sleep is a vital component of a healthy lifestyle, and it's essential for promoting long life. By making sleep a priority, you can improve your physical and mental health, enhance your quality of life, and potentially even extend your lifespan.

Effects of sleep deprivation on health and lifespan

Sleep deprivation can have a significant impact on an individual's health, both in the short-term and the long-term. Below are some of the potential effects:

- Impaired cognitive function: Sleep deprivation can affect attention, alertness, decision-making, and overall cognitive performance. It can also lead to memory problems and difficulty with learning.

- Mood disturbances: Lack of sleep can lead to irritability, mood swings, anxiety, and depression.

- Increased risk of accidents: Sleep deprivation can impair judgment and reaction time, leading to an increased risk of accidents and injuries.

- Weakened immune system: Chronic sleep deprivation can weaken the immune system, making individuals more susceptible to infections and illnesses.

- Weight gain: Sleep deprivation has been linked to an increased risk of obesity and weight gain, possibly due to alterations in hormone levels that control appetite and metabolism.

- Cardiovascular problems: Sleep deprivation has been linked to an increased risk of heart disease, high blood pressure, and stroke.

- Hormonal imbalances: Lack of sleep can disrupt the balance of hormones in the body, leading to a variety of health problems such as diabetes, infertility, and sexual dysfunction.

All the same, getting enough sleep is crucial for maintaining good health and well-being. I would recommend adults to have about 6-8 hours of sleep per night, while children and teenagers need even more. If you are experiencing sleep deprivation, it is important to address the underlying causes and take steps to improve your sleep habits.

Tips for improving sleep quality.

Sure, underlisted are some tips that may help you improve your sleep quality.

- Stick to a consistent sleep schedule: Try to go to bed and wake up at the same time every day, even on weekends. This helps regulate your body's internal clock and improve sleep quality.

- Create a relaxing bedtime routine: Develop a relaxing bedtime routine to signal to your body that it's time to wind down. This could include taking a warm bath, reading a book, or practicing relaxation techniques such as meditation or deep breathing.

- Make your bedroom conducive to sleep: Keep your bedroom quiet, cool, and dark. Invest in a comfortable mattress and pillows, and use blackout curtains or an eye mask if necessary.

- Limit caffeine and alcohol intake: Avoid caffeine and alcohol before bedtime as they can disrupt your sleep.

- Avoid electronic devices before bedtime: Blue light from electronic devices such as smartphones and tablets can interfere with your body's production of melatonin, a hormone that regulates sleep. Try to avoid using these devices for at least an hour before bedtime.

- Exercise regularly: Regular exercise can help improve sleep quality, but try to avoid exercising too close to bedtime as it can make it difficult to fall asleep.

- Manage stress: High levels of stress can make it difficult to fall asleep and stay asleep. Practice stress management techniques such as mindfulness, yoga, or journaling to help you relax.

Remember, improving your sleep quality may take time and effort, but it's worth it for the long-term benefits to your health and well-being.

Stress management

Effects of excessive stress on our health and life span.
Excessive stress can have negative effects on both our body and our overall life span. Below are some examples.

- Physical health: Stress can cause a wide range of physical health problems, including high blood pressure, heart disease, digestive problems, headaches, and weakened immune system, among others. Chronic stress can also lead to inflammation, which has been linked to a variety of chronic diseases.

- Mental health: Excessive stress can also take a toll on our mental health, leading to anxiety, depression, and other mental health disorders. It can also negatively impact our cognitive function, such as our ability to concentrate and remember information.

- Sleep problems: Stress can disrupt our sleep, making it difficult to fall asleep or stay asleep. This can lead to a host of other problems, including fatigue, irritability, and decreased productivity.

- Life span: Chronic stress can also affect our overall life span. Studies have shown that people who experience high levels of stress are at increased risk of premature death.

Stress Management tips for longlife

Certainly, below are some strategic tips for stress management that can help you live a long and healthy life

- Prioritize Self-Care: Set aside time for self-care activities that help you relax and unwind, such as meditation, yoga, or taking a relaxing bath. Prioritizing self-care can help you manage stress and improve your overall well-being.

- Get Enough Sleep: Lack of sleep can make you more susceptible to stress, so aim to get 7-9 hours of sleep per night. Establish a consistent bedtime routine, limit caffeine and alcohol, and create a relaxing sleep environment.

- Exercise Regularly: Exercise is a natural stress-reliever and can help boost your mood and energy levels. Aim to get at least 30 minutes of moderate exercise most days of the week.

- Practice Mindfulness: Mindfulness involves paying attention to the present moment without judgment. Regular mindfulness practice can help you manage stress, improve concentration, and promote relaxation.

- Connect with Others: Social support is an important buffer against stress. Make time to connect with friends and loved ones, whether it's through a phone call, text, or in-person visit.

- Seek Professional Help: If you're feeling overwhelmed or struggling to manage your stress, consider seeking help from a mental health professional. They can help you develop effective coping strategies and provide support and guidance as needed.

By implementing these strategies, you can better manage your stress levels and improve your overall well-being, which can help you live a long and healthy life.

There is no gainsaying, excessive stress can have a significant impact on our physical and mental health, as well as our overall quality of life and life span. It is important to find ways to manage stress effectively, such as through exercise, relaxation techniques, and seeking support from

*friends and family or a mental health
professional.*

Relaxation for health and Longevity

Relaxation and mindfulness techniques are incredibly important for living a long and healthy life. Both practices can help reduce stress, improve mental clarity, and promote a sense of calm and well-being. Here are some specific ways in which these techniques can benefit your health and longevity.

- Reducing stress: Chronic stress can lead to a variety of health problems, including high blood pressure, heart disease, and depression. Relaxation and mindfulness techniques, such as deep breathing, meditation, and yoga, can help reduce stress levels and promote relaxation.

- Improving sleep: Sleep is essential for overall health and longevity. Relaxation techniques can help you fall asleep faster and improve the quality of your sleep.

- Boosting the immune system: Chronic stress can weaken the immune system, leaving you more vulnerable to illness and disease. By reducing stress levels, relaxation and mindfulness techniques can help boost your immune system and improve your overall health.

- Improving mental clarity: Mindfulness techniques can help you become more aware of your thoughts and emotions, which can lead to greater mental clarity and focus. This can improve your overall cognitive function and help you stay sharp as you age.

- Promoting a sense of well-being: Finally, relaxation and mindfulness techniques can promote a sense of calm and well-being, which can improve your overall quality of life. By reducing stress and promoting relaxation, these techniques can help you feel happier and more content in your daily life.

In summary, relaxation and mindfulness techniques are essential for living a long and healthy life. By reducing stress, improving sleep, boosting the immune system, improving mental clarity, and promoting a sense of well-being, these practices can help you stay healthy and happy as you age.

Chapter Three

Diets: Improving good health and mortality rate

It is essential to take the below points to heart inorder to maintain good health and improve mortality rates.

- Soybeans

Soy is a food mainly consumed in Asia, including Japan where it is consumed as is after cooking (edamame) and especially in processed form, by fermentation (soy sauce, miso paste, nattō) or by coagulation of soy milk (tofu). It is an important source of isoflavones, molecules that have anticancer properties and are beneficial for good cardiovascular health. Consumption of isoflavones by Asians has been linked to a lower risk of breast and prostate cancer.

- Sugar

The Japanese, for example, consume relatively few sugars and starches, which partly explains the low prevalence of obesity-associated diseases such as ischemic heart disease and breast cancer. I strongly recommend we should learn from them.

- Green tea

The Japanese generally consume green tea with no added sugar. Prospective studies from Japan show that green tea consumption is associated with a lower risk of all-cause mortality and cardiac death.

Notable healthy diets to improve mortality rates.

There are several diets that have been linked to improved mortality rates. Some are mentioned and explained below.

- Mediterranean Diet: This diet emphasizes whole, minimally processed foods such as fruits, vegetables, whole grains, legumes, nuts, fish, and olive oil. It has been associated with reduced risk of heart disease, stroke, and certain cancers.

Mediterranean Diet breakdown

The Mediterranean diet is a traditional eating pattern that emphasizes plant-based foods, healthy fats, and lean proteins. Below is a breakdown of what the Mediterranean diet typically includes.

Fruits and vegetables: The Mediterranean diet emphasizes a variety of colorful fruits and vegetables, such as tomatoes, cucumbers, eggplant, peppers, spinach, kale, and citrus fruits.

Whole grains: Whole-grain bread, pasta, rice, and cereals are staples of the Mediterranean diet.

Legumes: Beans, lentils, chickpeas, and peas are a great source of protein and fiber in the Mediterranean diet.

Nuts and seeds: Almonds, walnuts, pistachios, and sunflower seeds are a common snack in the Mediterranean diet.

Olive oil: Olive oil is the primary source of fat in the Mediterranean diet, providing healthy monounsaturated fats.

Fish and seafood: Fatty fish such as salmon, tuna, and sardines are consumed frequently in the Mediterranean diet.

Poultry, eggs, and dairy: These foods are consumed in moderation in the Mediterranean diet.

Red meat and sweets: These are notably consumed sparingly in the Mediterranean diet.

In addition to the specific foods, the Mediterranean diet also emphasizes the following habits:

Eating meals with family and friends.

Enjoying food and eating slowly.

Using herbs and spices to flavor food instead of salt.

Drinking red wine in moderation (optional).

All the same, the Mediterranean diet is a healthy and sustainable eating pattern that has been associated with numerous health benefits, such as reducing the risk of heart disease, cancer, and cognitive decline.

- DASH Diet: The Dietary Approaches to Stop Hypertension (DASH) diet is rich in fruits, vegetables, whole grains, low-fat dairy, lean proteins, and nuts/seeds. It has been shown to lower blood pressure and reduce the risk of heart disease.

DASH Diet breakdown

The DASH (Dietary Approaches to Stop Hypertension) diet is a balanced, flexible and nutrient-rich eating plan designed to reduce blood pressure, prevent heart disease and improve overall health. The diet emphasizes a variety of foods from all food groups, while limiting or avoiding foods high in saturated fat, cholesterol, and sodium. Below is a breakdown of the DASH diet.

Fruits and Vegetables: Aim for 4-5 servings of fruits and 4-5 servings of vegetables per day. Choose a variety of colors and types, including leafy greens, berries, citrus fruits, sweet potatoes, carrots, and broccoli.

Grains: Choose whole grains such as brown rice, quinoa, oatmeal, whole wheat bread, and pasta. Aim for 6-8 servings per day.

Dairy: Choose low-fat or fat-free dairy products such as milk, yogurt, and cheese. Aim for 2-3 servings per day.

Protein: Choose lean protein sources such as chicken, fish, beans, nuts, and tofu. Aim for 6 or fewer servings per day.

Fats and oils: Use healthy fats such as olive oil, canola oil, avocado, and nuts. Limit saturated and trans fats.

Sweets and added sugars: Limit intake of sweets and added sugars to 5 or fewer servings per week.

Sodium: Aim for no more than 2,300 milligrams of sodium per day, or 1,500 milligrams per day if you have high blood pressure or are at risk for it.

In summary, the DASH diet encourages a balanced and varied diet rich in fruits, vegetables, whole grains, lean protein, and healthy fats, while limiting or avoiding foods high in saturated fat, cholesterol, and sodium. It is a healthy eating plan that can benefit everyone, especially those with high blood pressure or at risk for heart disease.

- Vegetarian/Vegan Diet: These diets exclude meat and other animal products, and emphasize plant-based foods. They have been linked to reduced risk of heart disease, diabetes, and certain cancers.

Vegetarian/Vegan Diet breakdown

A vegetarian diet is a plant-based diet that excludes meat, poultry, and fish, but may include eggs and dairy products. A vegan diet, on the other hand, is a plant-based diet that excludes all animal products, including eggs, dairy, and honey. Below is a breakdown of the different components of a vegetarian and vegan diet.

Protein: Vegetarians can get their protein from dairy products, eggs, legumes, nuts, seeds, and soy products. Vegans can get their protein from legumes, nuts, seeds, soy products, and grains.

Carbohydrates: Vegetarians and vegans can both get their carbohydrates from fruits, vegetables, whole grains, and legumes.

Fats: Both vegetarians and vegans can get their fats from nuts, seeds, avocado, olives, coconut, and plant-based oils like olive oil, coconut oil, and canola oil.

Vitamins and Minerals: Both vegetarians and vegans need to ensure they are getting adequate amounts of key vitamins and minerals like vitamin B12, vitamin D, calcium, iron, and zinc. Vegetarians can get these nutrients from dairy products and eggs, while vegans may need to supplement or consume fortified foods.

It's important to note that while vegetarian and vegan diets can be healthy, they can also be unhealthy if not planned properly. It's important to ensure that you are getting all of the necessary nutrients to maintain good health. Consulting a registered dietitian can be helpful in ensuring a well-balanced vegetarian or vegan diet.

- Nordic Diet: This diet emphasizes locally sourced foods such as berries, fish, whole grains, root vegetables, and canola oil. It has been associated with reduced risk of heart disease, stroke, and type 2 diabetes.

Nordic Diet breakdown

The Nordic Diet is a way of eating that emphasizes traditional foods commonly consumed in Denmark, Finland, Iceland, Norway, and Sweden. Below is a breakdown of the key components of the Nordic Diet.

Whole grains: The Nordic Diet emphasizes whole grains such as rye, oats, barley, and whole wheat. These grains are rich in fiber, vitamins, and minerals.

Berries: Berries such as blueberries, lingonberries, and cloudberries are a key component of the Nordic Diet. They are high in antioxidants and vitamins.

Fish: Fish such as salmon, herring, and mackerel are a main source of protein in the Nordic Diet. They are rich in omega-3 fatty acids, which have been linked to a reduced risk of heart disease.

Root vegetables: Root vegetables such as carrots, beets, and potatoes are commonly eaten in the Nordic Diet. They are a good source of fiber and vitamins.

Legumes: Legumes such as beans and lentils are also a part of the Nordic Diet. They are a good source of protein, fiber, and minerals.

Low-fat dairy: Low-fat dairy products such as milk, yogurt, and cheese are a part of the Nordic Diet. They are a good source of calcium and protein.

Herbs and spices: Herbs and spices such as dill, parsley, and cardamom are commonly used in Nordic cuisine. They add flavor to dishes without the need for salt or sugar.

In a nutshell, the Nordic Diet is a balanced and healthy way of eating that emphasizes whole, nutrient-dense foods.

- Japanese Diet: This diet is rich in fish, soy, vegetables, and fruit, and low in meat and dairy. It has been associated with reduced risk of heart disease, stroke, and certain cancers.

It's important to note that a healthy diet is just one aspect of a healthy lifestyle. Regular exercise, stress management, and avoiding tobacco and excessive alcohol consumption are also important factors in reducing mortality rates.

Japanese Diet breakdown

The traditional Japanese diet is known for being one of the healthiest diets in the world, with a focus on fresh, seasonal ingredients, fish, and vegetables. Here is a breakdown of the main components of a typical Japanese diet.

Rice: Rice is the staple food of the Japanese diet and is often eaten with every meal. It is usually steamed and served plain, but can also be mixed with other ingredients like vegetables or fish.

Fish: Fish is a key component of the Japanese diet, with a particular emphasis on fatty fish like salmon, mackerel, and tuna. Fish is often grilled or simmered in broth and served with rice and vegetables.

Vegetables: The Japanese diet is rich in vegetables, with a variety of leafy greens, root vegetables, and seaweed commonly eaten. Vegetables are often lightly cooked or served raw as part of a salad.

Soy products: Soy products like tofu, miso, and soy sauce are widely used in Japanese cuisine. These products are a good source of protein and are often used as a meat substitute.

Noodles: Noodles like udon and soba are commonly eaten in Japan, either as a soup or stir-fried with vegetables and meat.

Fruits: Fresh fruit is often eaten as a dessert or snack in Japan, with popular fruits including persimmons, oranges, and apples.

Tea: Tea is an important part of Japanese culture and is often served with meals. Green tea is the most popular type of tea in Japan and is believed to have numerous health benefits.

By all measures, the Japanese diet is low in saturated fat, high in fiber and antioxidants, and emphasizes a variety of fresh, whole foods.